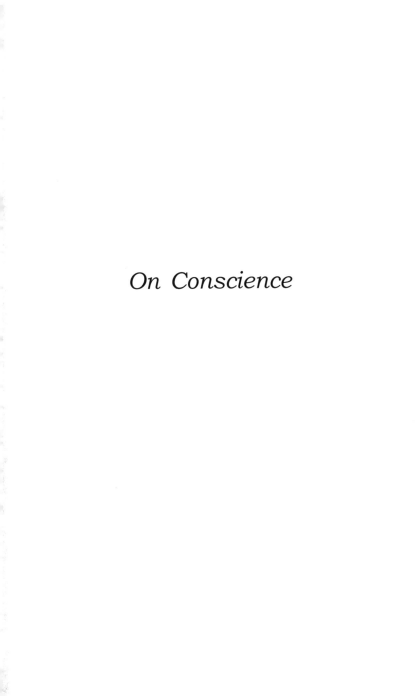

On Conscience

Bioethics & Culture Series
Edward J. Furton, General Editor

The National Catholic Bioethics Center was founded in 1972 to provide expert moral analysis and philosophical reflection in the fields of medicine, science, and technology. The NCBC seeks to promote and safeguard the dignity of the human person through research, education, consultation, and publishing. This mission, carried out for the sake of all people, is done with openness to the findings of science and with fidelity to the teachings of the Catholic Church. The NCBC includes among its key constituencies bishops and other clergy, health-care workers and academics, those who shape law and public policy, and numerous individuals who seek clarity on critical health-care issues affecting their families.

The National Catholic Bioethics Center
6399 Drexel Road
Philadelphia, PA 19151
www.ncbcenter.org

✠

On Conscience

TWO ESSAYS
BY JOSEPH RATZINGER

✠

THE NATIONAL CATHOLIC BIOETHICS CENTER
Philadelphia

IGNATIUS PRESS   San Francisco

The essays in this book were originally published by The Pope John XXIII Medical-Moral Research and Education Center (The Pope John Center), which changed its name in 1998 to The National Catholic Bioethics Center. The essays have been lightly edited for this edition, for punctuation and consistency of style.

"Conscience and Truth" originally appeared in *Catholic Conscience: Foundation and Formation* (Proceedings of the Tenth Bishops' Workshop), edited by Russell E. Smith © 1991 The Pope John Center, Braintree, Massachusetts. It was reprinted as *Conscience and Truth,* by Joseph Cardinal Ratzinger © 2000 The National Catholic Bioethics Center, Boston, Massachusetts.

"Bishops, Theologians, and Morality" first appeared in *Moral Theology Today: Certitudes and Doubts* (Proceedings of the Fourth Bishops' Workshop), edited by Donald G. McCarthy © 1984 The Pope John Center, St. Louis, Missouri.

National Catholic Bioethics Center
ISBN-10: 0-935372-48-2
ISBN-13: 978-0-935372-48-9
Library of Congress control no. 2005014048

Ignatius Press
ISBN-10: 1-58617-160-7
ISBN-13: 978-1-58617-160-5
Library of Congress control no. 2006920164

Contents

Foreword

This small volume contains two essays on conscience by Joseph Cardinal Ratzinger, now Pope Benedict XVI, written while he was Prefect of the Congregation for the Doctrine of the Faith. They should be put in context. They were both presented at workshops for bishops organized by The National Catholic Bioethics Center, then known as the Pope John XXIII Medical-Moral Research and Education Center. Since 1973, the center has organized workshops on medical-moral and bioethical topics, which have been attended by bishops from Canada, Mexico, Central America, the Caribbean, the Philippines, and the United States. These have always been fully and generously funded by the Knights of Columbus.

The NCBC bishops' workshops have always included topics of a more general theological or philosophical nature as well as topics dealing with quite specific issues such as abortion, sterilization, euthanasia, in vitro fertilization, and so forth. On two occasions, Cardinal Ratzinger presented the keynote address at these gatherings, first in 1984 and again in 1991.

In 1984, the workshop examined the relationship between the magisterium of the Church and theologians. In 1991, the workshop focused specifically on conscience and its exercise in particular circumstances. It is interesting that Benedict XVI's reflection on the working relationship between bishops and theologians was as concerned with the issue of conscience as was his address at the 1991 workshop, which dealt specifically with conscience. Although these addresses were separated by seven years and two different workshop themes, they both show that Cardinal Ratzinger's thought was profoundly occupied with the phenomenon of conscience. Consequently, the two essays together form a remarkably consistent theme for this little book.

The reflections of Benedict XVI show that contemporary debates over the nature of conscience have deep historical and philosophical roots, which can be traced back to the Enlightenment and beyond. The presentation of conscience as a subjective and, at the same time, infallible capacity for moral judgment manifests itself in the false opposition often posed between the magisterium as an external authority, imposing its decrees on hapless members of the Church, and the individual's personal, subjective conviction as to what is right. While Cardinal Ratzinger certainly accepts that one is bound to act in accord with a sure conscience, even if it is mistaken, he makes it clear that there must be sources for the judgment of conscience other than the subjective reflections of each individual. His wry humor is apparent as he remarks,

> It is strange that some theologians have difficulty accepting the precise and limited doctrine of papal infallibility, but see no problem in granting de facto infallibility to everyone who has a conscience. (66)

In these addresses, the Pope points out that there would be no moral norms at all if each person were able, with absolute certitude, to declare for himself what is morally right in every circumstance. What saves one from complete moral relativism are a number of factors necessary for morality: conscience, the shared experience of the community of which one is a part, reality itself, and finally what God has revealed of his will for us. Without these counterbalances to subjectivism, one faces the threat of a totalitarianism of the powerful arising from their own arbitrary decisions. This is precisely the theme Cardinal Ratzinger took up when he preached to the Cardinals before they went into the conclave that elected him Pope Benedict XVI. He warned them of their duty to protect the Church and the world from a "dictatorship of relativism."

When the only thing that determines what is morally right is one's individual, subjective judgment, then there is no overarching moral truth to which all are bound. In such a situation, those who have the greatest power can impose their positions on others, unchecked by any authority apart from themselves. Indeed, such an understanding of the infallibility of a subjective conscience would free from guilt, for example, even those who had committed unspeakable atrocities under German National Socialism (23). Pope Benedict is not prepared to ascribe such infallibility to subjective moral conviction. The nature of conscience is such, Cardinal Ratzinger has told us, that it could not possibly be blinded to the unspeakably heinous character of Nazi crimes. There would have to have been a degree of culpable silencing of conscience. No one can ultimately silence the voice of conscience that resides in each of us. No one can ultimately ignore the moral law that God Himself has inscribed on our hearts.

One of the characteristics of the scholarly work of Cardinal Ratzinger was always his ability to look at perennial problems from an unexpected perspective and address them in a novel way. He did this in his 1991 address when he spoke of the fundamental disposition to do good and avoid evil that is constitutive of every human being.

At least since the Middle Ages, the Catholic moral tradition has referred to this disposition as "synderesis," an unfamiliar, technical term that is used in virtually no other context than Catholic moral theology. In his 1991 address, Cardinal Ratzinger boldly and innovatively reached back to Plato and borrowed his term "anamnesis" to refer to this disposition (36). Plato taught that the Socratic method of teaching through questioning was a means of bringing the student to "remember" what he already knew. Cardinal Ratzinger believed that the concept of anamnesis communicated more effectively than synderesis the recalling of what constitutes our very being in terms of doing good and avoiding evil. This necessary recalling of our need to be disposed toward good and against evil helps avoid the subjectivism which he sees as so dangerous in our day.

In both these essays, and indeed in his homily before the conclave, Cardinal Ratzinger warned that the radical notion of a justifying, even though mistaken, conscience leads to a dictatorship of relativism, which invariably leads to a tyranny of the strong over the weak. That this danger is not simply a fancy of the Pope's imagination can be seen in the unbridled subjectivism of many U.S. Supreme Court decisions preceding and following the 1973 decision in *Roe v. Wade,* which legalized abortion. As the Court consistently repudiated challenges to this decision over the years, it adopted ever more sweeping articulations of a radical subjectivism, which reached its apotheosis in *Planned Parenthood v. Casey,* in the infamous "mystery" passage written by Justice Anthony Kennedy: "At the heart of liberty is the right to define one's own concept of existence, of meaning, of the universe, and of the mystery of human life."

In his repudiation of such a radical subjectivism as the basis for an understanding of conscience, Cardinal Ratzinger spoke in defense of human dignity and human rights in the same way in which Pope John Paul II did. In his encyclical *Evangelium vitae*, John Paul II wrote of the dangers to the weak and vulnerable arising from such subjectivism:

> To claim the right to abortion, infanticide and euthanasia, and to recognize that right in law, means to attribute to human freedom [or, in Cardinal Ratzinger's words, an infallible subjective conscience] a *perverse and evil significance*: that of an *absolute power over others and against others*. (n. 20, original emphases)

As mentioned above, one of the checks on a radical subjectivism leading to a so-called infallible conscience is reality itself. In his address to the 1991 bishops' workshop, Cardinal Ratzinger took a phrase of Cardinal John Henry Newman's, which is often used to justify a subjective conscience against teachings of the magisterium: "I would drink to the Pope, yes, but to conscience first" (29, paraphrased). Cardinal Ratzinger took the very quote that is often used to justify positions contrary to the Church's teaching on infallibility, to show that it can have no meaning apart from the Church's teaching on infallibility! It is to liberate and protect humanity that the Church exercises its infallibility in faith and morals, relying on the Holy Spirit, drawing on God's revelation, the experience and life of the community, and indeed reality itself. As Cardinal Ratzinger insisted, "The Church would betray, not only her own message, but the destiny of humanity if she were to renounce the guardianship of being and its moral message" (74). Being itself has a moral message precisely because it is a creation of God, who wills it and who inscribes it with its own purposefulness. Cardinal Ratzinger rightly points out that "When there is no God, there is no morality and, in fact, no mankind either" (74). Here he echoes the insightful words of the Fathers of the Second Vatican Council: "For without the Creator, the creature would disappear. ... When God is forgotten ... the creature itself becomes unintelligible" (*Gaudium et Spes*, n. 36).

Pope Benedict spoke of another guarantor of moral rectitude that prevents us from falling into the dangerous trap of a subjective conscience: the community that surrounds and shapes us and calls us out of ourselves. When thinking of Joseph Ratzinger, it is impossible not to think of the community that shaped and formed him, Catholic Bavaria, just as one must acknowledge the community that shaped and formed Karol Wojtyla, Catholic Poland. The abstraction of which Benedict speaks is not an abstraction. A personal reflection may perhaps be appropriate here.

The words of this foreword are written in Eichstätt, Bavaria, as I sit in a room in the guest house of St. Walburga's monastery, which was founded in 1083. The grand Baroque church of the monastery is built over the relics of the holy nun Walburga, sister of St. Willibald, the founding bishop of Eichstätt, who was consecrated by his uncle, St. Boniface, in 742. It is market day in the square below the monastery. Shoppers make their way over the cobblestones to the stalls of butchers, cheese merchants, and grocers. They mill beneath the fountain surmounted by a large statue of St. Willibald, while a brass band plays from the tower of the town hall. The bright music makes its way through my window along with the cool morning air.

Many years ago, Archbishop Joseph Ratzinger of Munich preached a retreat to the nuns of this monastery. The current abbess, Mother Franzeska, heard him as a young sister and still quotes him in her own meditations to her daughters. Across the valley is a long ridge out of which rises a hill crowned by a Baroque chapel honoring the Blessed Mother, Frauenberg, roughly translated "Marymount." Processions still make their way up the steep hills to the shrine, past wayside crucifixes and statues of saints nestled in the niches of houses and shops. The church bells in the town still ring the Angelus and mark the passing of each quarter hour and hour.

The townspeople are given to honesty, integrity, and hospitality. In the nearby village of Rebdorf, one is free to enter a field planted with strawberries and do one's own picking. There is a little metal box at the edge of the field where one simply drops one's coins for the berries picked—an unquestioned "honor system." Religious practices and countless proverbs constantly reinforce this sense of honesty, fairness, and uprightness. Herr Willibald Russer manages the conference center where I have often organized summer programs. He would set out a tray in which the participants could place their coins to pay for the beer or the soft drinks stacked in the refrigerator. He had not the slightest concern about the participants' honesty, as he would remind them, "*Mass und Gewicht, kommt vor Gottes Gericht,*" a little jingle meaning "Weight and measure come before God's throne of judgment." Be honest. God will judge.

Catholic Bavaria. It was this community that profoundly shaped and formed Joseph Ratzinger, a community in touch with reality, with God's revelation, with the living tradition of the Church.

Community is essential to the formation of conscience, Benedict reminds us in these essays. But Germans learned how the community itself can become disordered and not be the ultimate guarantor of moral rectitude if there is not a higher Guarantor still. As Cardinal Ratzinger told the Bishops gathered at the 1984 workshop, "everything depends on God, on a God who is Creator and on a God who has revealed Himself" (74). This is not a God over against the community, but One encountered precisely in the community. We also "need the community that can guarantee God, Whom no one on his own could dare bring into his life." This community is, of course, the Church.

Conscience, as a guarantor and an expression of human freedom, contributes to a sound morality formed by reality itself, by community, by God and His revelation, by one's own subjective perceptions and decisions. Conscience is such a radical guarantor of freedom that one would die before relinquishing it, as St. Thomas More and others have shown us (32). But it is also a bulwark and defense for the weak and the vulnerable who live among us. Regrettably, this understanding of conscience is almost unknown today. However, for the sake of a just social order, for the sake of human freedom and development, for the protection of the weak and the marginalized, it is an understanding that must be acquired once again. Pope Benedict calls us to anamnesis, to remembrance, not only of the moral law written in our hearts but also to a teaching on conscience that is true to our deepest traditions and to our own humanity.

JOHN M. HAAS
President
The National Catholic Bioethics Center

I

CONSCIENCE AND TRUTH

*Keynote address of the Tenth Bishops'
Workshop of the National Catholic Bioethics
Center, on "Catholic Conscience: Foundation
and Formation," February 1991*

In the contemporary discussion on what
constitutes the essence of morality and how it
can be recognized, the question of conscience
has become paramount, especially in the field
of Catholic moral theology. This discussion
centers on the concepts of freedom and norm,
autonomy and heteronomy, self-determination
and external determination by authority.

Conscience appears here as the bulwark of
freedom in contrast to encroachments of
authority on existence. In this, two notions of the
Catholic are set in opposition to each other. One
is a renewed understanding of the Catholic essence, which expounds Christian faith from the
basis of freedom and as the very principle of freedom itself. The other is a superseded,
"preconciliar" model, which subjects Christian
existence to authority, regulating life even in its

most intimate preserves, and thereby attempts to maintain control over people's lives. Morality of conscience and morality of authority, as two opposing models, appear to be locked in struggle with each other. Accordingly, the freedom of the Christian would be rescued by appeal to the classical principle of moral tradition: that conscience is the highest norm that man is to follow, even in opposition to authority. Authority—in this case, the magisterium—may well speak of matters moral, but only in the sense of presenting conscience with material for its own deliberation. Conscience would retain, however, the final word. Some authors reduce conscience in this, its aspect of final arbiter, to the formula "conscience is infallible."[1]

Nonetheless, at this point a contradiction can arise. It is, of course, undisputed that one must follow a certain conscience, or at least not act against it. But whether the judgment of conscience, or what one takes to be such, is always right—indeed, whether it is infallible—is another question. For if this were the case, it would mean that there is no truth—at least not in moral and religious matters, which is to say, in the areas that constitute the very pillars of our existence. For judgments of conscience can contradict each other. Thus there could be, at best, the subject's own truth, which would be reduced to the subject's sincerity. No door or window would lead from the subject into the broader world of being and human solidarity.

Whoever thinks this through will come to the realization that no real freedom exists then, and that the supposed pronouncements of conscience are but the reflection of social circumstances. This should necessarily lead to the conclusion that placing freedom in opposition to authority overlooks something. There must be something deeper if freedom and, therefore, human existence are to have meaning.

A Conversation on the Erroneous Conscience and First Inferences

It has become apparent that the question of conscience leads in fact to the core of the moral problem and thus to the question of man's existence itself. I would now like to pursue this question, not in the form of a strictly conceptual and therefore unavoidably abstract presentation, but by way of narrative, as one might say today—by relating, to begin with, the story of my own encounter with this problem.

I first became aware of the question with all its urgency in the beginning of my academic teaching. In the course of a dispute, a senior colleague, who was keenly aware of the plight of being Christian in our times, expressed the opinion that one should actually be grateful to God that He allows there to be so many unbelievers in good conscience. For if their eyes were opened and they became believers, they would not be capable, in this world of ours, of bearing the burden of faith with all its moral obligations. But as it is, since they can go another way in good conscience, they can still reach salvation.

What shocked me about this assertion was not in the first place the idea of an erroneous conscience given by God Himself in order to save men by means of such artfulness—the idea, so to speak, of a blindness sent by God for the salvation of those in question. What disturbed me was the notion it harbored that faith is a burden that can hardly be borne and that was, no doubt, intended only for stronger natures— faith almost as a kind of punishment—in any case, an imposition not easily coped with.

According to this view, faith would not make salvation easier but harder. Being happy would mean not being burdened with having to believe or having to submit to the moral yoke of the faith of the Catholic Church. The erroneous conscience, which makes life easier and marks a more human course, would then be the real grace, the normal way to salvation. Untruth, keeping truth at bay, would be better for man than truth. It would not be the truth that would set him free, but rather he would have to be freed from the truth. Man would be more at home in the dark than in the light. Faith would not be the good gift of the good God but instead an affliction.

If this were the state of affairs, how could faith give rise to joy? Who would have the courage to pass faith on to others? Would it not be better to spare them the truth or even keep them from it? In the last few decades, notions of this sort have discernibly crippled the disposition to evangelize. The one who sees the faith as a heavy burden or as a moral imposition is unable to invite others to believe. Rather, he lets them be, in the putative freedom of their good consciences.

The one who spoke in this manner was a sincere believer and, I would say, a strict Catholic, who performed his moral duty with care and conviction. But he expressed a form of experience of faith that is disquieting. Its propagation could only be fatal to the faith. The almost traumatic aversion many have to what they hold to be "preconciliar" Catholicism is rooted, I am convinced, in the encounter with such a faith, seen only as encumbrance. In this regard, to be sure, some very basic questions arise. Can such a faith actually be an encounter with truth? Is the truth about *God* and man so sad and difficult, or does truth not lie in the overcoming of such legalism? Does it not lie in freedom? But where does freedom lead? What course does it chart for us?

At the conclusion, we shall come back to these fundamental problems of Christian existence today, but before we do that, we must return to the core of our topic, namely, the matter of conscience. As I said, what unsettled me in the argument just recounted was first of all the caricature of faith I perceived in it. In a second course of reflection, it occurred to me further that the concept of conscience that it implied must also be wrong.

The erroneous conscience, by sheltering the person from the exacting demands of truth, saves him—thus went the argument. Conscience appears here not as a window through which one can see outward to that common truth that founds and sustains us all, and so makes possible through the common recognition of truth the community of wants and responsibilities. Conscience here does not mean man's openness to the ground of his being, the power of perception for what is highest and most essential. Rather, it appears as subjectivity's protective shell, into which man can escape and there hide from reality.

Liberalism's idea of conscience was, in fact, presupposed here: Conscience does not open the way to the redemptive road to truth—which either does not exist or, if it does, is too demanding. It is the faculty that dispenses with truth. It thereby becomes the justification for subjectivity, which would not like to have itself called into question. Similarly, it becomes the justification for social conformity. As mediating value between the different subjectivities, social conformity is intended to make living together possible. The obligation to seek the truth terminates, as do any doubts about the general inclination of society and what it has become accustomed to. Being convinced of oneself, as well as conforming to others, is sufficient. Man is reduced to his superficial conviction, and the less depth he has, the better for him.

What I was only dimly aware of in this conversation became glaringly clear a little later in a dispute among colleagues about the justifying power of the erroneous conscience. Objecting to this thesis, someone countered that if this were so, then the Nazi SS would be justified and we should seek them in heaven, since they carried out all their atrocities with fanatic conviction and complete certainty of conscience. Another colleague responded with utmost assurance that, of course, this was indeed the case: There is no doubting the fact that Hitler and his accomplices, who were deeply convinced of their cause, could not have acted otherwise. Therefore, the objective terribleness of their deeds notwithstanding, they acted morally, subjectively speaking. Since they followed their (albeit mistaken) consciences, one would have to recognize their conduct as moral and, as a result, should not doubt their eternal salvation.

Since that conversation, I knew with complete certainty that something was wrong with the theory of the justifying power of the subjective conscience—that, in other words, a concept of conscience that leads to such results must be false. Firm, subjective conviction and the lack of doubts and scruples that follow from it do not justify man.

Some thirty years later, in the terse words of psychologist Albert Görres, I found summarized the perceptions I was trying to articulate. The elaboration of his insights forms the heart of this address. Görres shows that the feeling of guilt, the capacity to recognize guilt, belongs essentially to the spiritual make-up of man. This feeling of guilt disturbs the false calm of conscience and could be called conscience's complaint against my self-satisfied existence. It is as necessary for man as the physical pain that signifies disturbances of normal bodily functioning. Whoever is no longer capable of perceiving guilt is spiritually ill, "a living corpse, a dramatic character's mask," as Görres says.[2]

> Monsters, among other brutes, are the ones without guilt feelings. Perhaps Hitler did not have any, or Himmler, or Stalin. Maybe Mafia bosses do not have any guilt feelings either, or maybe their remains are just well hidden in the cellar. Even aborted guilt feelings... All men need guilt feelings.[3]

By the way, a look into Sacred Scripture should have precluded such diagnoses and such a theory of justification by the errant conscience. In Psalm 19:12–13, we find the ever-worth-pondering passage, "But who can discern his errors? Clear thou me from my unknown faults." That is not Old Testament objectivism, but profoundest human wisdom. No longer seeing one's guilt, the falling silent of conscience in so many areas is an even more dangerous sickness of the soul than the guilt that one still recognizes as such. He who no longer notices that killing is a sin has fallen farther than the one who still recognizes the shamefulness of his actions, because the former is further removed from the truth and conversion.

Not without reason does the self-righteous man in the encounter with Jesus appear as the one who is really lost. If the tax collector with all his undisputed sins stands more justified before God than the Pharisee with all his undeniably good works (Luke 18:9–14), this is not because the sins of the tax collector were not sins or because the good deeds of the Pharisee were not good deeds. Nor does it mean that the good that man does is not good before God, or the evil, not evil or at least not particularly important.

The reason for this paradoxical judgment of God is shown precisely from our question. The Pharisee no longer knows that he too has guilt. He has a completely clear conscience. But this silence of conscience makes him impenetrable to God and men, while the cry of conscience that plagues the tax collector makes him capable of truth and love. Jesus can move sinners. Not hiding behind the screen of their erroneous consciences, they have not become unreachable for the change that God expects of them—of us. He is ineffective with the "righteous" because they are not aware of any need for forgiveness and conversion. Their consciences no longer accuse them but justify them.

We find something similar in St. Paul, who tells us that the pagans, even without the law, knew quite well what God expected of them (Romans 2:1–16). The whole theory of salvation through ignorance breaks apart with this verse: There is present in man the truth, which is not to be repulsed—that one truth of the Creator, which in the revelation of salvation history has also been put in writing. Man can see the truth of God from the fact of his creaturehood. Not to see it is guilt. It is not seen because man does not want to see it. The "no" of the will that hinders recognition is guilt. The fact that the signal lamp does not shine is the consequence of a deliberate looking away from that which we do not wish to see.[4]

At this point in our reflections, it is possible to draw some initial conclusions with a view toward answering the question regarding the essence of conscience. We can now say, It will not do to identify man's conscience with the self-consciousness of the "I," with its subjective certainty about itself and its moral behavior. On the one hand, this consciousness may be a mere reflection of the social surroundings and the opinions in circulation. On the other hand, it might also derive from a lack of self-criticism, a deficiency in listening to the depths of one's own soul.

This diagnosis is confirmed by what has come to light since the fall of Marxist systems in Eastern Europe. The noblest and keenest minds of the liberated peoples speak of an enormous spiritual devastation that appeared in the years of the intellectual deformation. They speak of a blunting of the moral sense, which is a more significant loss and danger than the economic damage that was done.

The new patriarch of Moscow stressed this poignantly in the summer of 1990. The power of perception of people who lived in a system of deception was darkened. The society lost the capacity for mercy, and human feelings were forsaken. A whole generation was lost for the good, lost for humane deeds. "We must lead society back to the eternal moral values," that is to say, open ears almost gone deaf, so that once again the promptings of God might be heard in human hearts. Error, the "erring" conscience, is only at first convenient. But then the silencing of conscience leads to the dehumanization of the world and to moral danger, if one does not work against it.

To put it differently, the identification of conscience with superficial consciousness, the reduction of man to his subjectivity, does not liberate but enslaves. It makes us totally dependent on the prevailing opinions, and debases these with every passing day. Whoever equates conscience with superficial conviction identifies conscience with a pseudo-rational certainty, a certainty that in fact has been woven from self-righteousness, conformity, and lethargy. Conscience is degraded to a mechanism for rationalization, while it should represent the transparency of the subject for the divine, and thus constitute the very dignity and greatness of man.

The reduction of conscience to subjective certitude betokens at the same time a retreat from truth. When the psalmist in anticipation of Jesus' view of sin and justice pleads for liberation from unconscious guilt, he points to the following relation: Certainly, one must follow an erroneous conscience. But the departure from truth that took place beforehand and now takes its revenge is the actual guilt, which first lulls man into false security and then abandons him in the trackless waste.

Newman and Socrates: Guides to Conscience

At this juncture, I would like to make a temporary digression. Before we attempt to formulate reasonable answers to the questions regarding the essence of conscience, we must first widen the basis of our considerations somewhat, going beyond the personal, which has thus far constituted our point of departure. To be sure, my purpose is not to try to develop a scholarly study on the history of theories of conscience, a subject on which different contributions have appeared just recently in fact.[5] I would prefer, rather, to stay with our approach thus far of example and narrative.

A first glance should be directed to Cardinal Newman, whose life and work could be designated a single great commentary on the question of conscience. Nor should Newman be treated in a technical way. The given framework does not permit us to weigh the particulars of Newman's concept of conscience. I would simply like to try to indicate the place of conscience in the whole of Newman's life and thought. The insights gained from this will hopefully sharpen our view of present problems and establish the link to history, that is, both to the great witnesses of conscience and to the origin of the Christian doctrine of living according to conscience.

When the subject of Newman and conscience is raised, the famous sentence from his letter to the Duke of Norfolk immediately comes to mind:

> Certainly, if I am obliged to bring religion into after-dinner toasts, (which indeed does not seem quite the thing), I shall drink—to the Pope, if you please,—still, to Conscience first, and to the Pope afterwards.[6]

In contrast to the statements of Gladstone, Newman sought to make a clear avowal of the papacy. And in contrast to mistaken forms of ultra-Montanism, Newman embraced an interpretation of the papacy, which is only then correctly conceived when it is viewed together with the primacy of conscience—a papacy not put in opposition to the primacy of conscience but based on it and guaranteeing it. Modem man, who presupposes the opposition of authority to subjectivity, has difficulty understanding this.

For him, conscience stands on the side of subjectivity and is the expression of the freedom of the subject. Authority, on the other hand, appears to him as the constraint on, threat to, and even negation of freedom. So, then, we must go deeper to recover a vision in which this kind of opposition does not obtain.

For Newman, the middle term—which establishes the connection between authority and subjectivity—is truth. I do not hesitate to say that truth is the central thought of Newman's intellectual grappling. Conscience is central for him because truth stands in the middle. To put it differently, the centrality of the concept *conscience* for Newman is linked to the prior centrality of the concept *truth,* and can only be understood from this vantage point. The dominance of the idea of conscience in Newman does not signify that he, in the nineteenth century, and in contrast to "objectivistic" neo-scholasticism, espoused a philosophy or theology of subjectivity. Certainly, the subject finds in Newman an attention that it had not received in Catholic theology perhaps since St. Augustine. But it is an attention in the line of Augustine and not in that of the subjectivist philosophy of the modem age.

On the occasion of his elevation to Cardinal, Newman declared that most of his life was a struggle against the spirit of liberalism in religion; we might add, also against Christian subjectivism, as he found it in the Evangelical movement of his time, which admittedly had provided him the first step on his lifelong road to conversion.[7]

Conscience for Newman does not mean that the subject is the standard vis-à-vis the claims of authority in a truthless world, a world that lives with a compromise between the claims of the subject and the claims of the social order. Much more than that, conscience signifies the perceptible and demanding presence of the voice of truth in the subject himself. It is the overcoming of mere subjectivity in the encounter of the inferiority of man with the truth from *God.* The verse Newman composed in 1833 in Sicily is characteristic: "I loved to choose and see my path; but now lead thou me on!"[8]

Newman's conversion to Catholicism was not for him a matter of personal taste or of subjective, spiritual need. He expressed himself on this even in 1844, on the threshold, so to speak, of his conversion: "No one can have a more unfavorable view than I of the present state of the Roman Catholics."[9] Newman was much more taken by the necessity to obey recognized truth than his own preferences, that is to say, even against his own sensitivity and bonds of friendship and ties due to similar backgrounds. It seems to me characteristic of Newman that he emphasized truth's priority over goodness in the order of virtues. Or, to put it in a way that is more understandable for us, he emphasized truth's priority over consensus, over the accommodation of groups.

I would say, when we are speaking of a man of conscience, we mean one who looks at things this way. A man of conscience is one who never acquires tolerance, well-being, success, public standing, and approval on the part of prevailing opinion at the expense of truth. In this regard Newman is related to Britain's other great witness of conscience, Thomas More, for whom conscience was not at all an expression of subjective stubbornness or obstinate heroism. He numbered himself, in fact, among those faint-hearted martyrs who only after faltering and much questioning succeed in mustering up obedience to conscience, mustering up obedience to the truth, which must stand higher than any human tribunal or any type of personal taste.[10]

Thus, two standards become apparent for ascertaining the presence of a real voice of conscience. First, conscience is not identical to personal wishes and taste. Second, conscience cannot be reduced to social advantage, to group consensus, or to the demands of political and social power.

Let us take a side look now at the situation of our day. The individual may not achieve his advancement or well-being at the cost of betraying what he recognizes to be true; nor may humanity. Here we come in contact with the really critical issue of the modern age. The concept of truth has been virtually given up, and replaced by the concept of progress. Progress itself "is" the truth. But through this seeming exaltation, progress loses its direction and becomes nullified. For if no direction exists, everything can just as well be regress as progress.

Einstein's relativity theory properly concerns the physical cosmos. But it seems to me to describe exactly the situation of the intellectual and spiritual world of our time. Relativity theory states that there are no fixed systems of reference in the universe. When we declare a system to be a reference point from which we try to measure the whole, it is we who do the determining. Only in such a way can we attain any results at all. But the determination could always have been done differently.

What we said about the physical cosmos is reflected in the second "Copernican revolution" regarding our basic relationship to reality. The truth as such, the absolute, the very reference point of thinking, is no longer visible. For this reason, precisely in the spiritual sense, there is no longer "up or down." There are no directions in a world without fixed measuring points. What we view to be direction is not based on a standard that is true in itself, but on our decision, and finally on considerations of expediency. In such a "relativistic" context, so-called ideological or consequentialist ethics ultimately becomes nihilistic, even if it fails to see this. And what is called conscience in such a worldview is, on deeper reflection, but a euphemistic way of saying that there is no such thing as an actual conscience, conscience understood as a "co-knowing" with the truth. Each person determines his own standards. And, needless to say, in general relativity, no one can be of much help to the other, much less prescribe behavior to him.

At this point, the whole radicality of today's dispute over ethics and conscience, its center, becomes plain. It seems to me that the parallel in the history of thought is the quarrel between Socrates-Plato and the Sophists, in which the fateful decision between two fundamental positions has been rehearsed. There is, on the one hand, the position of confidence in man's capacity for truth. On the other, there is a worldview in which man alone sets the standards for himself.[11] The fact that Socrates, the pagan, could become in a certain respect the prophet of Jesus Christ has its roots in this fundamental question. Socrates' taking up of this question bestowed on the way of philosophizing inspired by him a kind of salvation-historical privilege and made it an appropriate vessel for the Christian Logos. For with the Christian Logos we are dealing with liberation through truth and to truth.

If you isolate Socrates' dispute from the accidents of the time and take into account his use of other arguments and terminology, you begin to see how much his is the same dilemma we face today. Giving up the idea of man's capacity for truth leads first to pure formalism in the use of words and concepts. Again, the loss of content, then and now, leads to a pure formalism of judgment. In many places today, for example, no one bothers any longer to ask what a person thinks. The verdict on someone's thinking is ready at hand as long as you can assign it to its corresponding, formal category: conservative, reactionary, fundamentalist, progressive, revolutionary. Assignment to a formal scheme suffices to render unnecessary coming to terms with the content.

The same thing can be seen in more concentrated form in art. What a work of art says is indifferent. It can glorify God or the devil. The sole standard is that of formal, technical mastery.

We have now arrived at the heart of the matter. Where contents no longer count, where pure praxeology takes over, technique becomes the highest criterion. This means, though, that power becomes the preeminent category, whether revolutionary or reactionary. This is precisely the distorted form of being-like-God of which the account of the fall speaks. The way of mere technical skill, the way of sheer power, is imitation of an idol, and not expression of one's being made in the image and likeness of God. What characterizes man as man is not that he asks about the "can" but about the "should," and that he opens himself to the voice and demands of truth.

It seems to me that this was the final meaning of the Socratic search, and it is the profoundest element in the witness of all martyrs. They attest to the fact that man's capacity for truth is a limit on all power and a guarantee of man's likeness to God. It is precisely in this way that the martyrs are the great witnesses of conscience, of that capability given to man to perceive the "should" beyond the "can" and thereby render possible real progress, real ascent.

Systematic Consequences:
The Two Levels of Conscience

Anamnesis

After all these ramblings through intellectual history, it is finally time to arrive at some conclusions, that is, to formulate a concept of conscience. The medieval tradition was right, I believe, in according two levels to the concept of conscience. These levels, though they can be well distinguished, must be continually referred to each other.[12] It seems to me that many unacceptable theses regarding conscience are the result of neglecting either the difference or the connection between the two. Mainstream scholasticism expressed these two levels in the concepts "synderesis" and "conscientia."

The word *synderesis (synteresis)* came into the medieval tradition of conscience from the stoic doctrine of the microcosm.[13] It remained unclear in its exact meaning, and for this reason became a hindrance to a careful development of this essential aspect of the whole question of conscience. I would like, therefore, without entering into philosophical disputes, to replace this problematic word with the much more clearly defined Platonic concept of anamnesis. It is not only linguistically clearer and philosophically deeper and purer, but anamnesis above all also harmonizes with key motifs of biblical thought and the anthropology derived from it.

The word *anamnesis* should be taken to mean exactly that which Paul expressed in the second chapter of his Letter to the Romans:

> When Gentiles who have not the law do by nature what the law requires, they are a law to themselves, even though they do not have the law. They show that what the law requires is written on their hearts, while their conscience also bears witness ... (2: 14–15)

The same thought is strikingly amplified in the great monastic rule of Saint Basil. Here we read:

> The love of God is not founded on a discipline imposed on us from outside, but is constitutively established in us as the capacity and necessity of our rational nature.

Basil speaks in terms of "the spark of divine love which has been hidden in us," an expression that was to become important in medieval mysticism.[14] In the spirit of Johannine theology Basil knows that love consists in keeping the commandments. For this reason, the spark of love, which has been put into us by the Creator, means this: "We have received interiorly beforehand the capacity and disposition for observing all divine commandments ... These are not something imposed from without." Referring everything back to its simple core, Augustine adds, "We could never judge that one thing is better than another, if a basic understanding of the good had not already been instilled in us."[15]

This means that the first so-called ontological level of the phenomenon conscience consists in the fact that something like an original memory of the good and true (they are identical) has been implanted in us, that there is an inner ontological tendency within man, who is created in the likeness of God, toward the divine. From its origin, man's being resonates with some things and clashes with others. This anamnesis of the origin, which results from the god-like constitution of our being, is not a conceptually articulated knowing, a store of retrievable contents. It is, so to speak, an inner sense, a capacity to recall, so that the one whom it addresses, if he is not turned in on himself, hears its echo from within. He sees: That's it! That is what my nature points to and seeks.

The possibility for and right to mission rest on this anamnesis of the Creator, which is identical to the ground of our existence. The gospel may, indeed must, be proclaimed to the pagans, because they themselves are yearning for it in the hidden recesses of their souls (see Isaiah 42:4). Mission is vindicated, then, when those addressed recognize in the encounter with the word of the gospel that this indeed is what they have been waiting for.

In this sense Paul can say that the gentiles are a law to themselves—not in the sense of the modern liberal notions of autonomy, which preclude transcendence of the subject, but in the much deeper sense that nothing belongs less to me than I myself. My own "I" is the site of the profoundest surpassing of self and contact with him from whom I came and toward whom I am going.

In these sentences, Paul expresses the experience which he had had as missionary to the gentiles and which Israel may have experienced before him in dealings with the "god-fearing." Israel could have experienced among the gentiles what the ambassadors of Jesus Christ found reconfirmed. Their proclamation answered an expectation. Their proclamation encountered an antecedent basic knowledge of the essential constants of the will of God, which came to be written down in the commandments, which can be found in all cultures, and which can be all the more clearly elucidated the less an overbearing cultural bias distorts this primordial knowledge. The more man lives in "fear of the Lord" (consider the story of Cornelius, especially Acts 10: 34–35), the more concretely and clearly effective this anamnesis becomes.

Again, let us take a formulation of St. Basil. The love of God, which is concrete in the commandments, is not imposed on us from without, the church father emphasizes, but has been implanted in us beforehand. The sense for the good has been stamped upon us, as Augustine puts it. We can now appreciate Newman's toast first to conscience and then to the pope. The pope cannot impose commandments on faithful Catholics because he wants to or finds it expedient. Such a modern, voluntaristic concept of authority can only distort the true theological meaning of the papacy. The true nature of the Petrine office has become so incomprehensible in the modern age no doubt because we think of authority only in terms that do not allow for bridges between subject and object. Accordingly, everything that does not come from the subject is thought to be externally imposed.

But the situation is really quite different according to the anthropology of conscience, of which we have tried to come to an appreciation in these reflections. The anamnesis instilled in our being needs, one might say, assistance from without so that it can become aware of itself. But this "from without" is not something set in opposition to anamnesis but is ordered to it. It has maieutic function, imposes nothing foreign, but brings to fruition what is proper to anamnesis, namely, its interior openness to the truth.

When we are dealing with the question of faith and church, whose radius extends from the redeeming Logos over the gift of creation, we must, however, take into account yet another dimension, which is especially developed in the Johannine writings. John is familiar with the anamnesis of the new "we," which is granted to us in the incorporation into Christ (one body, that is, one "I" with him). In remembering, they knew him, as the Gospel has it in a number of places.

The original encounter with Jesus gave the disciples what all generations thereafter receive in their foundational encounter with the Lord in baptism and the Eucharist, namely, the new anamnesis of faith, which unfolds, like the anamnesis of creation, in constant dialogue between *within* and *without*. In contrast to the presumption of gnostic teachers, who wanted to convince the faithful that their naive faith must be understood and applied much differently, John could say, You do not need such instruction; as anointed ones (baptized ones) you know everything (see 1 John2: 20).

This does not mean a factual omniscience on the part of the faithful. It does signify, however, the sureness of the Christian memory. This Christian memory, to be sure, is always learning, but proceeding from its sacramental identity, it also distinguishes *from within* between what is a genuine unfolding of its recollection and what is its destruction or falsification. In the crisis of the Church today, the power of this recollection and the truth of the apostolic word are experienced in an entirely new way, where (much more so than hierarchical direction) it is the power of memory of the simple faith that leads to the discernment of spirits.

One can comprehend the primacy of the pope and its correlation to Christian conscience only in this connection. The true sense of the teaching authority of the pope consists in his being the advocate of the Christian memory. The pope does not impose from without. Rather, he elucidates the Christian memory and defends it. For this reason the toast to conscience indeed must precede the toast to the pope, because without conscience there would not be a papacy. All power that the papacy has is power of conscience. It is service to the double memory on which the faith is based—and which again and again must be purified, expanded, and defended against the destruction of memory that is threatened by a subjectivity forgetful of its own foundation, as well as by the pressures of social and cultural conformity.

Conscientia

Having considered this first, essentially ontological level of the concept of conscience, we must now turn to its second level—that of judgment and decision, which the medieval tradition designates with the single word *conscientia,* conscience. Presumably this terminological tradition has not insignificantly contributed to the diminution of the concept of conscience. Saint Thomas, for example, designates only this second level as *conscientia.* For him it stands to reason that conscience is not a *habitus,* that is, a lasting ontic quality of man, but *actus,* an event in execution. Thomas, of course, assumes as given the ontological foundation of anamnesis *(synderesis).* He describes anamnesis as an inner repugnance to evil and attraction to the good.

The act of conscience applies this basic knowledge to the particular situation. It is divided, according to Thomas, into three elements: recognizing (*recognoscere*), bearing witness (*testificari*), and finally judging (*iudicare*). One might speak of an interaction between a function of control and a function of decision.[16] Thomas sees this sequence according to the Aristotelian tradition's model of deductive reasoning. But he is careful to emphasize what is peculiar to this knowledge of moral actions whose conclusions do not come from mere knowing or thinking.[17]

Whether something is recognized or not depends too on the will, which can block the way to recognition or lead to it. It is dependent, that is to say, on an already formed moral character, which can either continue to deform or be further purified.[18] On this level, the level of judgment (*conscientia* in the narrower sense), it can be said that even the erroneous conscience binds. This statement is completely intelligible from the rational tradition of scholasticism. No one may act against his convictions, as St. Paul had already said (Romans14:23). But this fact—that the conviction a person has come to certainly binds in the moment of acting—does not signify a canonization of subjectivity. It is never wrong to follow the convictions one has arrived at—in fact, one must do so. But it can very well be wrong to have come to such askew convictions in the first place, by having stifled the protest of the anamnesis of being.

The guilt lies then in a different place, much deeper—not in the present act, not in the present judgment of conscience, but in the neglect of my being that made me deaf to the internal promptings of truth.[19] For this reason, criminals of conviction like Hitler and Stalin are guilty. These crass examples should not serve to put us at ease but should rouse us to take seriously the earnestness of the plea, "Free me from my unknown guilt" (Psalm 19:13).

Epilogue:
Conscience and Grace

At the end there remains the question with which we began: Is not the truth, at least as the faith of the Church shows it to us, too lofty and difficult for man? Taking into consideration everything we have said, we can respond as follows:

Certainly, the high road to truth and goodness is not a comfortable one. It challenges man. Nevertheless, retreat into self, however comfortable, does not redeem. The self withers away and becomes lost. But in ascending the heights of the good, man discovers more and more the beauty that lies in the arduousness of truth, which constitutes redemption for him.

But not everything has yet been said. We would dissolve Christianity into moralism if no message that surpasses our own actions became discernible. Without many words, an image from the Greek world can show us this. In it we can observe simultaneously both how the anamnesis of the Creator extends from within us outward toward the Redeemer, and how everyone may see him as redeemer, because he answers our own innermost expectations.

I am speaking of the story of the expiation of Orestes' sin of matricide. Orestes had committed the murder as an act of conscience. This is designated by the mythological language of obedience to the command of the god Apollo. But now Orestes finds himself hounded by the Furies, or *Erinyes,* who are mythological personifications of conscience and who, from a deeper wellspring of recollection, reproach him, declaring that his decision of conscience, his obedience to the "saying of the gods," was in reality guilt. The whole tragedy of man comes to light in this dispute of the "gods," that is to say, in this conflict of conscience. In the holy court, the white stone of Athena leads to Orestes' acquittal, his sanctification, in the power of which the *Erinyes* are transformed into *Eumenides,* the spirits of reconciliation. Atonement has transformed the world.

The myth, while representing the transition from a system of blood vengeance to the right order of community, signifies much more than just that. Hans Urs von Balthasar expressed this "more" as follows: "Calming grace always assists in the establishing of justice, not the old graceless justice of the *Erinyes* period, but that which is full of grace..."[20] This myth speaks to us of the human longing that conscience's objectively just indictment—and the attendant destructive, interior distress it causes in man—not be the last word. It thus speaks of an authority of grace, a power of expiation that allows the guilt to vanish and makes truth at last truly redemptive. It is the longing for a truth that does not just make demands of us, but also transforms us through expiation and pardon. Through these, as Aeschylus puts it, "guilt is washed away,"[21] and our being is transformed from within, beyond our own capability.

This is the real innovation of Christianity: The Logos, the truth in person, is also the atonement, the transforming forgiveness that is above and beyond our capability and incapability. Therein lies the real novelty on which the larger Christian memory is founded, and which indeed, at the same time, constitutes the deeper answer to what the anamnesis of the Creator expects of us.

Where this center of the Christian message is not sufficiently expressed and appreciated, truth becomes a yoke that is too heavy for our shoulders, from which we must seek to free ourselves. But the freedom gained thereby is empty. It leads into the desolate land of nothingness and disintegrates of itself. Yet the yoke of truth in fact became "easy" (Matthew 11: 30) when the Truth came, loved us, and consumed our guilt in the fire of his love. Only when we know and experience this from within will we be free to hear the message of conscience with joy and without fear.

II

Bishops, Theologians, and Morality

*Keynote address of the Fourth Bishops'
Workshop of the National Catholic Bioethics
Center, on "Moral Theology Today:
Certitudes and Doubts," February 1984*

The word "moral" is slowly beginning to regain a place of honor. For it is becoming ever more clear that we *should* not do everything we can do. It is becoming ever more evident that the peculiar sickness of the modern world is its failings in morality. Recently, a Russian author said:

> Mankind today, with his dread of missiles, is like a man who lives in continual fear that his house will be burned down. He can think of nothing else but how to prevent the arson. In so doing, he does not notice that he has cancer. He will not die of arson, but by the inner decomposition of his body brought on by the alien organism of the cancer.

So mankind today, says this author, is in danger of being ruined from within, by his own moral decay. But instead of struggling against this life-threatening disease, he stares as though hypnotized at the external danger, which is only a by-product of his own inner moral disease.

Still, it has become a rather common observation that the value placed upon technical expertise is out of all proportion when compared to the scant attention paid to moral development. Today we seem to know more about how to *build* bombs than how to judge whether it is moral to *use* them. This lack of proportion paid to morality is the key question of our day. Therefore, the renewal of morality is not just some rearguard action of a zealot opposed to progress, but *the* critical question on which any real progress will depend.

Thus, in this workshop we will not be dealing with disputed points that are of interest only to the Church; rather, we are standing at the very point where the Church goes beyond herself. It is precisely when we look at her moral message that we can see that the Church is not some kind of club for the satisfaction of social or even personal ideal needs. Rather, we see that she performs an essential service right in the midst of the turmoil that society is going through. She is not, in the first place, some kind of "moral institution." That is how they tried to describe her and to justify her existence in the period of the Enlightenment. Nevertheless, she *does* have something to do with the moral resources of humanity. We could call these moral resources the most important raw material we have for human existence now, and for making possible a future in which it will still be worthwhile to be a person.

The question posed by my theme might be formulated like this: What contribution can the Church make toward forging a balance between external progress and morality? What can she do, not just to keep herself in existence, but to open up once again the moral resources of humanity? One might go so far as to say the Church will survive only if she is in a position to help mankind overcome this hour of trial. In order to do this, she must show herself as a moral power. And she must do this in two ways: She must set standards, and she must awaken both the will and the power of people to respond to these standards. In this context the question takes on a particular shape, namely, how can bishops work together with theologians, the bishops being charged with the transmission of the faith and the theologians being charged with the dialogue between the world of faith and the mind-set of the world at large?

It would be too facile to answer these questions with a few tactical formulas to produce a satisfactory agreement between those who are responsible for the decisions and the experts, even though it is so important to work out and make use of such practical rules. But it is not at *all* so easy to reproduce mechanically the general structural relationship between the competence to make decisions and expert knowledge. Each maintains its own form through the particular character of the matter involved. So it is necessary before searching for rules for collaboration between bishops and moral theologians, first of all, to reflect—at least in very general outline—on the question of the sources and the method of moral knowledge. How can we arrive at moral knowledge at all? How do we arrive at correct moral judgments?

The Four Sources of Moral Knowledge and Their Problems

Reduction to "Objectivity"

When we come now to the question we have posed for ourselves concerning the method of moral knowledge, we see very clearly the poverty of the modern world about which we have already spoken: its lack of ideas when faced with the moral problem, the underdevelopment of moral reason as compared with calculating reason. A mark of modern society is specialization, which also includes a division of labor. This results in competence to acquire knowledge: In the individual fields of human knowledge and action, the particular specialist is competent who, in the process of our ever-expanding and precise knowledge, manages to get an overview and an experience of a specific sector. But are there specialists in the field of morality, which does not admit of division of labor, when they all proceed each in his own way?

A division of labor in the area of knowledge presumes a quantification of the object of knowledge. One might think here of Henry Ford's famous assembly line. Every worker performs a specific task in the overall construction of the Model T. No one worker can build a whole car, much less design one, or even know how the mechanism functions.

One can divide and distribute only that which has become a quantity. The success of modern science is based on the translation of the reality we encounter into quantitative measures. In this way the world becomes measurable and technologically exploitable. But could we not say that the crisis of humanity in our times finds its roots in this method and in its increasing domination in all aspects of human life? Calculation, which in turn is subject to what is quantitative, is the method of what is not free. It works when we are dealing with what can be calculated, ordered and necessary. It is good for building cars.

If morality, however, is the area of freedom, and if its norms are laws of freedom, then inevitably these laws will not be sufficient for us: They must leave us perplexed in the face of that which is truly human. A simple answer suggests itself here. Perhaps freedom is only an illusion, the remains of an old dream of humanity from which, for better or for worse, we must separate ourselves. Does not everything point to the fact that man, caught up in the physical and biological net of reality, is thoroughly determined? Must not a complete enlightenment lead to a situation in which, even in mankind, morality will be replaced by technique, that is, by a correct ordering and combination of predetermined elements that will then yield the desired result?

And so there emerges the thought of calculating human behavior to analyze the predetermined state that is proper and fundamental to man, and so to discover a formula for happiness and survival. Statistics and planning together provide the new "morality" with which man prepares his way into the future. All moral rules, which man could then calculate, would thus be directed to those ends that man himself has in mind for humanity. Just as man designs technical tools for his own purposes, so in the area of morality he imposes his own goals on the laws of nature.

But here the decisive question remains open: Who determines the goals? Who plans the future of man? Granted there are many who are powerful who would gladly arrogate this right to themselves, no one of us has the right to do so. Who then could have the right to oblige all men to pursue one particular goal or another? At this point we must postpone attempts to answer the question of the sources of morality, but this is not to imply that it is either resolved or unessential.

A second question now emerges: If there are ends that man must pursue, how does he know them? It should be clear that we cannot reduce moral knowledge to some model of knowledge in general, understood as the calculation and combination of known measures that are demonstrable because of their repetition.

Obviously, it cannot be disputed that a good amount of useful data about mankind and the world can, nevertheless, be gathered in this way. But since human behavior is not at all so easy to repeat or reproduce identically in others, any attempt to subject human behavior to a purely scientific analysis encounters sooner or later an insurmountable limitation: namely, the limitations of humanity itself, which is after all what we are discussing.

Only at the price of ignoring what is precisely human could the question of morality be analyzed in the ordinary way of human knowing. The fact that this is actually being attempted in various quarters today is the great inner threat to mankind today. The tree of knowledge, from which man eats in this case, does not give the knowledge of good and evil, but rather blinds man to discerning the difference between them. Man will not return to paradise through such blindness, because it is not based on a purer humanity but on the rejection of humanity.[1]

Subjectivity and Conscience

We see, then, that in the question of morality there cannot be experts in the same way that there can be experts in microelectronics or computer science. Plato realized that when he said that a person cannot express "with scholastic words" what the word "good" means.[2] But in what other way can we learn it?

There are a number of suggestions here that must be examined in order, but briefly. It is only in the convergence of the various ways that we can find the way itself.

To begin with, there is today a broadly accepted alternative to the complete objectification of moral knowledge, whose shortcomings we have just seen. In one sector of modern thinking we have the strange situation where man, faced with both the greatness and the limitations of quantitative analysis, tries to overcome the distinction between the subject and object. We can calculate the world since, and to the extent that, we make it an "object."

Opposed to this "objective," which is what can be studied by science, there remains the "subjective," the world of the incalculable and the free. In this division of the world, religion and morality are relegated to the world of the subjective. They are subjective in the sense that they cannot be analyzed by science or placed within the generally valid criteria of ordinary knowledge. In this view the subjective really does exist, although the ultimate analysis of it is up to the individual's imagination to decide.

Obviously, in such a reduction of morality to the subjective it becomes impossible to address the objective concerns of our day that demand a moral answer.[3] To that extent, this approach to the problem is losing favor today. Still, in practical life and especially in the discussion within the Church itself, it still plays an important role, insofar as here the subjection of morality to the area of the subjective has become linked with the long Christian tradition of the teaching on conscience.

Conscience is understood by many as a sort of deification of subjectivity, a rock of bronze on which even the magisterium is shattered. It is said that in light of the conscience, no other cases apply. Conscience appears finally as subjectivity raised to the ultimate standard.

We will have to examine this question in closer detail, as it already touches directly the precise theme of my essay. For the moment, however, I note that conscience is presented as one source of moral knowledge, that is to say, a personal, primitive knowledge of good and evil which appears in the individual man as a source of his ability to make moral judgments.

The Will of God and His Revelation

If we follow a little further the pathway of *conscience* as we find it in the tradition, then we encounter another fundamental element in the moral area. The idea of conscience cannot be separated in its history from the idea of the responsibility of man before God.

To a great extent, conscience expresses the thought of a kind of co-knowledge of man with

God, and precisely from here there emerges the absoluteness with which conscience asserts its superiority over any and all authorities. The history of morality is inseparably linked with the history of thought about God. As far as the fixed character of the natural laws is concerned, morality means the free "yes" given by one will to another, in this case, the conformity of man to the will of God and the consequent correct perception of things as they really are. As an ultimate source of morality, then, we have to take into consideration the process of how God makes His desires for mankind known, how one acquires knowledge of the divine commandments in which the special ends of man and the world become clear. If such objective morality is based on revelation, then immediately the next question arises: How can one know revelation as revelation? How can revelation be identified as such?

The Community as a Source of Morality

Here we meet with another factor that has played and still plays an extremely important role in the working out of various moral theories. The Latin word *mores* without any distinction contains meanings that we have learned to distinguish carefully: *Mores* are the habits, customs, and lifestyle of a people, practically what we would call today "the American way of life" or the "California style." At the same time, alongside the totality of life habits, the word also has a specifically moral meaning.

When St. Augustine, for example, wrote *De moribus ecclesiae catholicae et de moribus Manichaeorum*, it was not a question of comparative morality in today's sense. Rather, in making a comparison between the form of life of the Catholic Church, her total lifestyle, and that of the Manichaeans, he goes on to distinguish two distinct types of morality within the broader context of lifestyle. Likewise, in the language of the Council of Trent, the formula *fides et mores* does not simply mean faith and morals in today's sense of the terms, but rather in the broader sense in which the customs of the life of the Church, including moral order in the strict sense, are understood.

In this use of language something very important appears: "morality" is not an abstract code of norms for behavior, but presupposes a community way of life within which morality itself is clarified and is able to be observed. Historically considered, morality does not belong to the area of subjectivity, but is guaranteed by the community and has a reference to the community. In the lifestyle of a community the experience of generations is stored up: experiences of things that can build up a society or tear it down, how the happiness of an individual and the continuity of the community as a whole can be brought together in a balanced way, and how that equilibrium can be maintained.

Every morality needs its "we," with its prerational and suprarational experiences, in which not only the analysis of the present moment speaks, but also the wisdom of the generations converges.

A crisis in morality occurs in a community when new areas of knowledge emerge with which the current life patterns cannot cope, to the point that what up until then appeared as supportive and proven appears now as insufficient or, indeed, contradictory, or as an obstacle to the new knowledge and reality. Then the question arises, How can the community find a new way of life that will once more make possible a common moral existence for life and for the world itself? It remains true that morality needs a "we" and that it requires a link with the experience of past generations and with the primitive wisdom of humanity.

And so we return to the question from which we began, namely, the problem of revelation. We can make this assertion: The various concrete community experiences of different races and peoples are valuable as signposts for human behavior, but by themselves cannot be considered sources for morality. It is impossible in the long run to have a society that lives, as it were, only as a reaction from what is negative and evil. If a society wishes to survive, it must to a certain extent return to the primitive virtues, to the basic, standard models of humanity.

Still, it is certainly possible for important areas of life in a society to become corrupt, so that the predominant custom of men and women does not guide but seduces, as in a society with the custom of cannibalism, slavery, or dependence on drugs. An individual can rely on his own experience and on the common historical experiences only to a limited degree. In history, therefore, morality was never based exclusively on experience and custom. Its unconditional character could not be understood except in reference to the unconditional character of God's will: In the last analysis, morality was founded on a divine revelation of will, out of which alone a community could emerge and in accord with which the survival of the community as such was guaranteed.

I must leave aside at this point a series of questions that really ought to be asked, so that I can return to my particular theme. Despite the fragmentary nature of these reflections so far, we can nevertheless see that the faith of the Church is in agreement with the fundamental traditions of humanity on several points. Christian faith is also convinced that God alone can be the measure of man and that only the divine will can unconditionally oblige man. Christian faith is further convinced that revelation situates us in the community life model of a "we" whose nature and direction cannot be explained simply in terms of the human will alone.

Clearly, the Christian looks at this "we," whose customs constitute the proximate source of moral knowledge, not simply in terms of his own local society, but in terms of a new society, which can be explained only through revelation, which transcends all local societies (it is "catholic"), and which subordinates them to the dictates of the divine will that are addressed to them all.

With this as a context, one can experience what morality is by seeking in the first place the *mores ecclesiae:* Thus the person who is by virtue of his office responsible for the form of life of the Church—the bishop—in Catholic tradition bears the principal responsibility for teaching Christians morals as well as faith. It also means that in the area of morality those who have the greatest right to speak are those who live according to the deepest essence of the Church to the most profound degree—the saints.

But with these remarks I have moved on too quickly. I simply wanted to note the fact that we are still working toward our theme, even though it may seem that our aim has disappeared in the individual points of this reflection. Perhaps it would be good at this point to sum up what we have seen, so that then, as far as we can, we can move on to the concrete implications of all of this.

We have located four sources of morality. If taken in isolation from each other, each leaves several questions unanswered. But when they are taken in combination, then the path of moral knowledge opens up before us. If, on one hand, we have to conclude that authentic morality cannot be constructed on the basis of an examination of the concrete world alone, still morality must be concerned with objective morality, since moral behavior must do justice to truth. It is in this way that *reality*—and reason, which knows and explains reality—is without a doubt an irreplaceable source of morality.

As a second source, we spoke of *conscience*. The *wisdom of tradition* is a third source, embodied in a living "we," an active community which for the Christian is concretely realized in the new community of the Church.

Finally, we saw that all these sources lead to true morality when *the will of God* is present. For in the final analysis, only the will of God can establish the boundary between good and evil, which is something different from the boundary between what is useful or not or what is proved and what is unknown. The Catholic Church sees an important confirmation of her teaching in the fact that within her these elements interpenetrate and illuminate each other. Her teaching brings conscience to expression. Conscience is seen to be valid precisely because it incorporates the inner truth of things in accord with reality, which is after all the voice of the Creator.

These three things—objectivity, tradition, and conscience—in turn point to the divine commandments.

These commandments on one hand constitute the basis of the Church's teaching, they form consciences and make reality intelligible.

On the other hand, because they correspond to reality as perceived by conscience, they are for their part able to be confirmed as true revelations of the divine will.

Second Principal Problem: Conscience and Objectivity

No doubt it might be observed that what I have just said is an idealization of a reality which in fact is not all that harmonious. A number of nuances would have to be added in order to be more realistic. Two main objections, related to the first two of the four sources of morality, tend now to arise.

There is the rather common impression that the Church is not in a position to respond in a correct manner to reality in today's world. Instead of listening to the language of reality, she is immovably chained to antiquated points of view that she tries to impose on men. Right here a conflict arises between the bishop and the expert. In many ways this conflict appears to be a conflict between a doctrine that is distant from reality and an exact understanding of current reality.

The second objection comes from the area of conscience. The consciences of many Christians are by no means in harmony with many expressions of the Church's magisterium. Indeed, it often seems that the conscience is that which gives dissent some legitimacy.

So, then, if we wish to arrive at a clear position with regard to the function of the bishop as teacher of morality and his relationship to the experts in moral theology, then it is necessary, if only in rough outline, to look into the two questions that have arisen:What is conscience? And how can one learn which form of behavior corresponds to things as they really are, to reality, and is thus moral behavior in the meaningful sense of the term?

What Is Conscience and How Does It Speak?

When one speaks of conscience today, three principal streams of thought come to mind.[4] We have already touched on the first of these. For conscience asserts the right of subjectivity, which can in no way be measured objectively. But in response there immediately arises the objection, Who establishes such an absolute right of subjectivity? It may indeed have a relative right, but in really important cases must not that right be sacrificed to an objective common good of the highest level?

It is strange that some theologians have difficulty accepting the precise and limited doctrine of papal infallibility, but see no problem in granting de facto infallibility to everyone who has a conscience. In fact, it is not possible to assert an absolute right for subjectivity as such.

Conscience also signifies in some way the voice of God within us. With this notion the completely inviolable character of the conscience is established: In conscience we have a case that would be above any human law. The fact of such a direct bond between God and man gives man an absolute dignity. But then the question arises, Does God speak to men in a contradictory manner? Does He contradict Himself? Does He forbid one person, even to the point of martyrdom, to do something that He allows or even requires of another?

It is clear that it is not possible to justify the equation of the individual judgments of conscience with the voice of God. Conscience is not an oracle, as Robert Spaemann rightly noted.

We now encounter a third meaning: Conscience is the superego, the internalization of the will and the convictions of others who have formed us and have so impressed their will on us that it no longer speaks to us externally, but rather from deep within our inner self. In this sense, conscience would not be a real source of morality at all, but only the reflection of the will of another, an alien guide within ourselves. Conscience would not then be an organ of freedom, but an internalized slavery from which man would logically have to free himself in order to discover the breadth of his real freedom.

Even though one might explain many individual expressions of conscience in this way, this theory cannot stand completely.

On one hand we find children who, before they are formally educated, react spontaneously against injustice. They give a spontaneous "yes" to what is good and true, which precedes any educational interventions—interventions that often enough only darken them or crush them rather than let them grow. On the other hand, there are mature men and women in whom one finds a freedom and an alertness of conscience that sets itself against what has been learned or what is commonly done. Such a conscience has become an inner sense of what is good, a kind of remote control to guide man through what he has been taught.

What is the real position of conscience? I wish to make my own what Robert Spaemann has said about it: Conscience is an organ, not an oracle.[5] It is an organ because it is something that for us is a given, which belongs to our essence, and not something that has been made outside of us. But because it is an organ, it requires growth, training, and practice. I find the comparison that Spaemann makes with speech is very fitting in this case. Why do we speak? We speak because we have learned to speak from our parents. We speak the language that they taught us, although we realize there are other languages, which we cannot speak or understand. The person who has never learned to speak is mute. And yet language is not an external conditioning that we have internalized, but rather something that is properly internal to us. It is formed from outside, but this formation responds to the given of our own nature: that we can express ourselves in language.

Man is as such a speaking essence, but he becomes so only insofar as he learns speech from others. In this way we encounter the fundamental notion of what it means to be a man: Man is "a being who needs the help of others to become what he is in himself."[6]

We see this fundamental anthropological structure once again in conscience. Man is in himself a being who has an organ of internal knowledge about good and evil. But for it to become what it is, it needs the help of others. Conscience requires formation and education. It can become stunted, it can be stamped out, it can be falsified so that it can only speak in a stunted or distorted way. The silence of conscience can become a deadly sickness for an entire civilization.

In the Psalms we meet from time to time the prayer that God should free man from his hidden sins. The Psalmist sees as his greatest danger the fact that he no longer recognizes them as sins and thus falls into them in apparently good conscience. Not being able to have a guilty conscience is a sickness, just as not being able to experience pain is a sickness, again as Spaemann says.[7] And thus one cannot approve the maxim that everyone may always do what his conscience allows him to do: In that case the person without a conscience would be permitted to do anything.[8] In truth it is his fault that his conscience is so broken that he no longer sees what he as a man should see.

In other words, included in the concept of conscience is an obligation, namely, the obligation to care for it, to form it and educate it. Conscience has a right to respect and obedience in the measure in which the person himself respects it and gives it the care which its dignity deserves. The right of conscience is the obligation of the formation of conscience. Just as we try to develop our use of language and we try to rule our use of rules, so must we also seek the true measure of conscience so that finally the inner word of conscience can arrive at its validity.

For us this means that the Church's magisterium bears the responsibility for correct formation. It makes an appeal, one can say, to the inner vibrations its word causes in the process of the maturing of conscience. It is thus an oversimplification to put a statement of the magisterium in opposition to conscience. In such a case I must ask myself much more. What is it in me that contradicts this word of the magisterium? Is it perhaps only my comfort? My obstinacy? Or is it an estrangement through some way of life that allows me something which the magisterium forbids and that appears to me to be better motivated or more suitable simply because society considers it reasonable? It is only in the context of this kind of struggle that the conscience can be trained, and the magisterium has the right to expect that the conscience will be open to it in a manner befitting the seriousness of the matter.

If I believe that the Church has its origins in the Lord, then the teaching office in the Church has a right to expect that it, as it authentically develops, will be accepted as a priority factor in the formation of conscience. There corresponds to this, then, an obligation of the magisterium to speak its word in such a way that it will be understood in the midst of conflicts of values and orientations. It must express itself in such a way that an inner resonance of its word may be possible within the conscience, and this means more than just an occasional declaration of the highest level.

Here we need what Plato was referring to when he said the good cannot be known scholastically, but only after regular familial discussion can the notion of the good spring into the soul like light springing from a small spark.[9] This constant "familial discussion" within the Church must build up the community conscience—those who try to express their word in the teaching office, as well as those who wish to learn that word from within themselves.

Nature, Reason, and Objectivity

Thus, we have already arrived at the other point on which I want to touch: The word of the magisterium is for many Christians today no longer plausible because its reasonableness and objectivity are no longer transparent. The magisterium is accused of setting out from an outdated understanding of reality. Like the old

Stoics, the magisterium argues from "nature." But this expression, "nature," has been completely overlooked by the entire metaphysical age.

At first, this so-called naturalism of the magisterial tradition was seen in opposition to the personalism of the Bible. The opposition of nature and person as a basic pattern for argumentation was at the same time seen as an opposition between philosophical and biblical tradition. Still, it has now long been recognized that there is no such thing as a pure "biblicism," and that even "personalism" has its own philosophical aspects.

Today we see almost the direct opposite movement: The Bible has to a great extent vanished from the modern works in moral theology. In its place, a tendency toward a particularly strong rational analysis has become dominant, together with the assertion of the autonomy of morals, which is based neither on nature nor on the person, but on historicity and future-oriented models of social behavior.

One must try to discover what is socially compatible and what serves the building of a future human society. The "reality" on which "objectivity" is based is seen no longer as a nature that precedes man, but rather in the world that he himself has structured, which one may now simply analyze and from which one may extrapolate what the future will bring.[10] Here we come up against the real reason why Christianity today (not only in the area of the moral) to a great extent lacks direct plausibility. As we have already seen, as a result of the philosophical change introduced by Kant, the division of reality into subjective and objective has become dominant.

The objective is not simply reality in itself, but reality only inasmuch as it is the object of our thought and is thus measurable and can be calculated. The subjective, for its part, eludes "objective" explanation. This means, however, that the reality we encounter speaks only the language of human calculation, but has within itself no moral expression. The constantly expanding radical forms of the theory of evolution lead to the same conclusion, though from a different starting point: The world presupposes no reason; what is reasonable in it is the result of a combination of accidents whose ongoing accumulation developed a kind of necessity.

According to such a viewpoint, the world contains no meaning, but only goals, which are posited by evolution itself.[11] If the world is thus a montage of static appearances, then the highest moral directive it can then give to man is that he himself should be engaged in some kind of montage of the future, and that he himself should direct everything according to what he reckons is useful. The norm thus lies always in the future: In this view the greatest possible betterment of the world is the only moral commandment.

In contrast, the Church believes that in the beginning was the Logos and that therefore being itself bears the language of the Logos—not just mathematical, but also aesthetical and moral reason. This is what is meant when the Church insists that "nature" has a moral expression. No one is saying that biologism should become the standard of man. That viewpoint has been recommended only by some behavioral scientists.

The Church professes herself the advocate of the reason of creation and practices what she means when she says, "I believe in God, the Creator of Heaven and Earth." There is a reason for being, and when man separates himself from it totally and recognizes the reason only of what he himself has made, then he abandons what is precisely moral in the strict sense. In some way or another we are beginning to realize that materiality contains a spiritual expression, and that it is not simply for calculation and use. In some way we see that there is a reason that precedes us, which alone can keep our reason in balance and can keep us from falling into external unreason.

In the last analysis, the language of being, the language of nature, is identical with the language of conscience.[12] But in order to hear that language, it is necessary, as with all language, to practice it. The organ for this, however, has become deadened in our technical world. This is why there is a lack of plausibility here. The

Church would betray, not only her own message, but the destiny of humanity if she were to renounce the guardianship of being and its moral message. In this sense she may be opposed to what is "plausible," but at the same time she stands for the most profound claims of reason. It becomes obvious here that reason too is an organ and not an oracle. And reason too requires training and community.

Whether a person is able to attribute reason to being and to decipher his own moral dimension depends on whether he answers the question about God. If the Logos of the beginning does not exist, neither can there be any Logos in things. What Kolakowski discovered, then, becomes emphatically true: When there is no God, there is no morality and, in fact, no mankind either.[13] In this sense, in the deeper analysis, everything depends on God, on a God who is Creator and on a God who has revealed Himself. For this reason, once again, we need the community that can guarantee God, Whom no one on his own could dare bring into his life.

Even Abraham, our father in faith, was not being completely innovative when he introduced monotheism 2,000 years before Christ. Even that primitive society already cherished its belief in the divine.

The question of God, which is the central point, is not a question for specialists. The perception of God is precisely that simplicity which the specialists can never monopolize, but rather which can be perceived only by maintaining a simplicity of vision. Perhaps we find it so difficult today to deal with the essence of humanity because we have ceased being capable of simplicity.[14]

Therefore, morality requires not the specialist, but the witness. The position of the bishop as teacher rests on this: He teaches not what he himself has discovered. But he witnesses to the life wisdom of faith, in which the primitive wisdom of humanity is cleansed, maintained, and deepened. Through contact with God, depending on how perceptive the conscience is, this primitive human knowledge becomes a real vehicle of communication with truth by means of the communion it shares with the conscience of the saints and with the knowledge of Jesus Christ.

Naturally, it does not follow from this that scientific work regarding the criteria of morality and specialized knowledge in this area have become unnecessary. Since conscience requires training, since tradition must be lived and must develop in times of change, and since moral behavior is a response to reality and therefore requires a knowledge of reality—for all these reasons the observation and study of reality as well as the traditions of moral thought are important.

To put it another way, to seek a thorough knowledge of reality is a fundamental commandment of morality. It was not without reason that the ancients placed *prudence* as the first cardinal virtue: They understood it to mean the willingness and the capacity to perceive reality and respond to it in an objective manner.[15]

Applications

Now that we have considered all of this, we can formulate the essential tasks of both bishop and specialized theologian in moral questions, and from this will automatically emerge the rules for their working together in a correct manner.

The Bishop as Teacher of Morality

The bishop is a witness to the *mores ecclesiae catholicae,* to those rules of life that have grown up in the common experience of the believing conscience in the struggle with God and with historical reality. As a witness, the bishop must in the first place know this tradition in its foundations, its content, and its various stages. One can only bear witness to what one knows. The knowledge of the essential moral tradition of the faith is therefore a fundamental demand of the episcopal office.

Since it is a question of a tradition that comes from conscience and speaks to conscience, the bishop himself must be a man of a seeing and listening conscience. He must strive, in living the *mores ecclesiae catholicae,* to see that his own personal conscience is sharpened. He must know morality not second- but first-hand. He must not simply pass on a tradition, but bear witness to what has become for himself a credible and proven lifestyle.

Setting out from such a personal knowledge of the moral word of the Church, he must attempt to remain in discussion with those experts who seek the correct application of the simple words of faith to the complicated reality of a particular time. He must therefore be prepared to become a learner and a critical partner of the experts. He must learn to see where it is a question of the knowledge of new realities, new problems, new possibilities for understanding and so for maturing and cleansing the moral heritage. He must be critical when expert science forgets its own boundaries or reduces morality to a simple specialization.

The Tasks of the Moral Theologian

On the basis of our reflections so far, we might define the tasks of the moral theologian in the following manner:

As a theologian, the moral theologian also finds his starting point in the *mores ecclesiae catholicae,* which he researches and which, in their essential link with what is Catholic, he distinguishes. And so he also tries to recognize in the *mores* that which is specifically moral and constant and to understand them in a unified way in the total context of the faith. He seeks the *ratio fidei.*

He then brings this reason of faith in a critical way into dialogue with the reason and the plausibility of the particular time. He helps toward the understanding of the moral demands of the Gospel in the particular conditions of his day and so serves the formation of conscience. In this way he serves also the development, purification, and deepening of the moral message of the Church.

Above all, the moral theologian will also take up the new questions that new developments and relationships pose for the traditional norms. He will attempt to know precisely the objective components of such discussions (for example, the technology of armaments, economic problems, and medical developments) in order to work out the best way to pose the questions and so arrive at the relationship with the constants of the moral tradition of the faith. In this sense he stands in critical dialogue with the moral evaluations of society, and in all this he helps the teaching office of the Church present its moral message in the particular time.

The Relationship between
Bishop and Theologian

From our reflections on the individual tasks, it is now possible to derive the fundamental rules for the relationship between teaching office and expert.

The teaching office depends on the specialized knowledge of the experts and must let itself be thoroughly informed by them about the content of the matter in question before making an utterance regarding new problems. The teaching office must therefore not be too hasty in taking up a position regarding questions that are not yet clarified, nor must it apply its binding statements beyond what the principles of tradition permit.

On the other hand, the teaching office of the Church must defend man against himself to prevent his destruction, even if this means opposing the philosophy of an entire epoch. For example, in a period in which the world thinks of itself only as a product and as an end, the teaching office of the Church must continually try to get nature to be recognized as creation in its defense of the unborn. There is an obligation to inform, an obligation to respect the boundaries of universally binding moral statements, and an obligation to witness. The moral catechesis must go beyond that which can be determined with certainty and should offer models of behavior in concrete circumstances (casuistry).

But it seems important to me clearly to distinguish between these cases and the specific moral teaching. I have the impression that the regular and un-nuanced introduction of cases into the specific moral statement, or likewise the failure to distinguish between them, has contributed to discrediting the moral teaching of the Church in our century in a substantial way.

But the task of the moral theologian is not simply to be in service to the teaching office. It also stands in dialogue with the ethical questions of the time and contributes, through the development of models of behavior, to the process of the formation of conscience. As regards the magisterium, his task is to precede it: He goes before it, noticing new questions, gathering knowledge of their objective content, and preparing answers. The moral theologian likewise accompanies the magisterium and follows it, bringing its pronouncements into the dialogue of his time and relating the basic lines of the discussion to concrete situations.

Criticism of the Magisterium:
Its Rules and Limits

Today, interest in the relationship between the episcopal magisterium and scientific theology is concentrated above all on the question, Can the moral theologian criticize the teaching office?

After what we have said about the structure of moral expression and its relationship to specialized science, we must make some distinctions. First of all, we must apply here what the Second Vatican Council said about the steps of assent, and in like manner the stages of criticism, with regard to Church teaching. Criticism may be framed according to the level and demands of the magisterial teaching. It will be all the more helpful when it fills in a lack of information, clarifies shortcomings of the linguistic or conceptual presentation, and at the same time deepens the insight into the limits and range of the particular teaching.

In the light of our reflection, on the other hand, we see that it is not for the expert himself to draw up norms or to annul the norms, perhaps by setting up factions or pressure groups. As we have seen, norms can only be witnessed to, but not produced or annulled by some calculated analysis. When this happens, the peculiar nature of morality itself is misunderstood. Therefore, dissent can have meaning only in the area of casuistry, not in the specific area of norms. The most important thing in the relationship between the magisterium and moral theology appears to me, in the last analysis, to lie in what Plato recommends as the path to moral knowledge: in "regular familial discussion," a discussion in which we must all learn to become more and more hearers of the biblical word, vitally addressed and directed to the *mores ecclesiae catholicae.*

Notes

CONSCIENCE AND TRUTH

1. This thesis was apparently first proposed by J. G. Fichte: "Conscience does [not] and cannot err," because it is "itself judge of all conviction," which "recognizes no higher judge over itself. It is the ultimate authority and cannot be appealed" (*System der Sittenlehre* [1798], III, 15; reprinted in *Fichtes Werke,* vol. 4, ed. I. M. Fichte [Berlin: de Gruyter, 1971], 174). See H. Reiner, "*Gewissen,*" in J. Ritter and K. Grunder, eds.: *Historisches Wörterbuch der Philosophie* 3 (1974): 574–592, here 586. Kant had already previously formulated the counterarguments. They appear in more depth in Hegel, for whom conscience "as formal subjectivity…[is] always on the verge of changing into evil" (see Reiner, "Gewissen"). Nevertheless, the thesis of the infallibility of conscience is at present again in the ascendancy in popular theological literature. I find a—in a certain respect—mediating position in E. Schockenhoff, *Das umstrittene Gewissen* (Mainz, Germany: 1990), which expressly reckons with the possibility that conscience can miss its mark "by going astray of the other requirement of the oral law, the mutual recognition of the free rational being" (139). Schockenhoff, however—relying on [F. X.] Linsenmann—rejects talk of an erring conscience: "In view of the quality of conscience as such, there is no sense in speaking of error, because there is no higher observation point from which error could be ascertained" (136). Why

not? Is there no truth concerning the good [that is] accessible to all of us in common? To be sure, the point is then so significantly nuanced that finally, in the end, it is even less clear to me why the concept of the erring conscience should be untenable. Helpful here is M. Honecker, *Einfuhrung in die theologische Ethik* (Berlin: 1990), l38ff.

2. A. Görres, "Schuld und Schuldgefahle," in *Internationale katholische Zeitschrift "Communio"* 13 (1984): 434.

3. Ibid., 442.

4. See Honecker, *Einfuhrung in die theologische Ethik,* 130.

5. Besides the important article of Reiner and the work of Schockenhoff on new studies (already cited), see A. Laun, *Das Gewissen: Oberste Norm sittlichen Handelns* (Innsbruck, Austria: 1984) and his *Aktuelle Probleme der Moraltheologie* (Vienna, Austria: 1991), 31–64; J. Gründel, ed., *Das Gewissen: Subjektive Willkür oder oberste Norm?* (Dusseldorf, 1990); and a summary overview, "Gewissen," by K. Golser, in H. Rotter and G. Virt, eds., *Neues Lexikon der christlichen Moral* (Innsbruck, Austria: Tyrolia, 1990), 278–286.

6. Newman to the Duke of Norfolk, December 27, 1874, in *The Works of Cardinal Newman: Difficulties of Anglicans,* vol. 2 (Westminster, MD: Christian Classics, 1969), 261; see J. Honore, *Newman: Sa Vie et sa Pensée* (Paris: 1988), 65, and I. Ker, *John Henry Newman: A Biography* (Oxford, UK: Oxford University, 1990), 688ff.

7. See C. Dessain, *John Henry Newman: A Biography*, 3rd edition (Oxford, UK: Oxford University, 1980); and G. Biemer, *John Henry Newman: Leben und Werk* (Mainz, Germany: Grünewald, 1989).

8. From the famous poem "Lead Kindly Light," in Newman, *Verses on Various Occasions* (London:

Longmans, 1888); cf. Ker, *Newman,* 79, and Dessain, *Newman,* 33–34.

9. Newman to J. Keble, December 29, 1844, in *Correspondence of J. H. Newman with J. Keble and Others: 1839–1845* (London: 1917), 364; see also 351 and Dessain, *Newman,* 79.

10. See P. Berglar, *Die Stunde des Thomas Morus,* 3rd edition (Olten, Switzerland: Walter, 1981), 155ff.

11. Regarding the debate between Socrates and the Sophists, see J. Pieper, "Missbrauch der Sprache —Missbrauch der Macht," in *Uber die Schwierigkeit, heute zu glauben* (Munich, Germany: 1974), 255–282; and *Kummert euch nicht um Sokrates* (Munich: 1966). A penetrating treatment of the question of the truth as the center of Socratic searching is found in R. Guardini, *The Death of Socrates* (New York: 1948).

12. A short summary of the medieval doctrine of conscience can be found in Reiner, "Gewissen," 582–583.

13. See E. von Ivanka, *Plato Christianus* (Einsiedeln, Switzerland: Johannes, 1964), 315–351, especially 320–321.

14. Basil, *Regulae fusius tractatae,* Resp. 2,1: PG 31, 908.

15. Augustine, *De Trinitate* VIII, 3 (4), PL 42, 949.

16. See Reiner, *"Gewissen,"* 582; Aquinas, *Summa theologiae* I, q. 79, a. 13; and Aquinas, *De Ver,* q. 17, a. 1.

17. See the careful study of L. Melina, *La conoscenza morale: Linee di reflessione sul commento di San Tommaso all'Etica Nicomachea* (Rome: Città Nuova Editrice, 1987), 69ff.

18. In reflecting on his own inner experience in the decades following his conversion, St. Augustine elaborated fundamental insights into the essence of freedom and morality concerning the relationships

between knowledge, will, emotion, and inclination through habit. See the excellent presentation of P. Brown, *Augustine of Hippo: A Biography* (New York: Dorset, 1986), 146–157.

19. That this precisely is also the position of St. Thomas Aquinas is shown by I. G. Belmans in his extremely enlightening study, "Le paradoxe de la conscience erronee d'Abélard à Karl Rahner," *Revue Thomiste* 90 (1990): 570–586. He shows how, with the publication of Sertillanges' book on St. Thomas in 1942, a then widely adopted distortion of Thomas's doctrine of conscience takes hold, which—to put it simply—consists in the fact that only the *Summa theologiae* I–II, q.19, a. 5 ("Must one follow an erroneous conscience?") is cited, and the following article, a. 6 ("Is it sufficient to follow one's conscience in order to act properly?"), is simply ignored. That means imputing the doctrine of Abelard to Thomas, whose goal was in fact to overcome Abelard. Abelard had taught that the crucifiers of Christ would not have sinned if they had acted from ignorance. The oniy way to sin consists in acting against conscience. The modern theories of the autonomy of conscience can appeal to Abelard but not to Thomas.

20. Hans Urs von Balthasar, *Glory of the Lord: A Theological Aesthetics,* vol. 4: *The Realm of Metaphysics in Antiquity* (San Francisco, CA: Ignatius Press, 1989), 121.

21. Aeschylus, *Eumenides*, 2nd edition, ed. G. Murray (Oxford, UK: Oxford University, 1955), 280–281; von Balthasar, *Glory of the Lord* 4: 121.

BISHOPS, THEOLOGIANS, AND MORALITY

1. For the problems addressed here, see F. H. Tenbruck, *Die unbewaltigten Sozialwissenschaften oder die Abschaffung des Menschen* (Graz, Austria: 1984).

2. Plato, Letter 7, 341c; see R. Spaemann, *Moralische Grundbegriffe* (Munich, Germany: Beck, 1982).

3. This issue is very nicely set forth by W. Heisenberg, *Der Teil und das Ganze* (Munich, Germany: Piper, 1969), 116–130 and 279–295.

4. See R. Spaemann, *Moralische Grundbegriffe,* 73–84. Also helpful is A. Laun, *Das Gewissen: Oberste Norm sittlichen Handelns* (Innsbruck, Austria: 1984).

5. Spaemann, *Moralische Grundbegriffe,* 81.

6. Ibid., 79.

7. Ibid., 80.

8. Ibid., 83.

9. Plato, Letter 7, 341c.

10. For these issues, see the painstaking presentation by J. Finnis, *Fundamentals of Ethics* (Washington, DC: Georgetown University Press, 1983). Also enlightening is F. Ricken, "Kann die Moralphilosophie auf die Frage nach dem 'Ethischen' verzichten?" in *Theol. Phil.* 59 (1984): 161–77.

11. For a treatment of this problem area, see Spaemann and R. Löw, *Die Frage Wozu? Geschichte und Wiederentdeckung des teleologischen Denkens* (Munich, Germany: Piper, 1981).

12. We learn much about the idea of Nature in its relation to morality in H. Ratner, "Nature, Mother and Teacher: Her Norms," *Listening: Journal of Religion and Culture* 18 (1983): 185–219.

13. L. Kolakowski, *Falls es keinen Gott gibt* (Munich, Germany: Piper, 1982): 173–191; see also 82. It would be profitable in this connection to reflect again on Ludwig Wittengenstein's "Aussagen zu den ethischen Satzen" in his *Tractatus logico-philosophicus* (German/English; London: 1961), especially 6.41: "Der Sinn der Welt muss ausserhalb ihrer liegen..."; 6.42: "Darum kann es auch keine Sätze der Ethik

geben..."; and 6.422: "Also muss diese Frage nach den Folgen einer Handlung belanglos sein."

14. Kolakowski has formulated the gist of this issue from a unique perspective, saying, "One must take this opportunity to repeat the question posed by Erasmus and his colleagues: Why is the Gospel so understandable for everyone except those spirits who are ruined by theological speculation? This pertains to all sacred texts, whether they were written or orally handed on. Believers understand the language of the Saints in their proper role, i.e, as an aspect of adoration" (*Falls es keinen Gott gibt,* 157).

15. See J. Pieper, *Das Viergespann* (Munich, Germany: Kosel, 1964), 15–64.